Flavorful Fortified

Food

Recipes to Enrich Life

Digna Cassens, MHA, RD &
Linda S. Eck Mills, MBA, RD, FADA

First Edition, June 2012
Copyright 2012 Digna Cassens, MHA, RD, & Linda S. Eck Mills, MBA, RD, FADA

This recipe book is a collection of well tried and tested recipes previously published in various articles, journals and manuals by the authors.

Published by:

    Cassens Associates – Diversified Nutrition Management Systems
    PO Box 581
    La Habra, CA 90633
    dignacassens@gmail.com
                    &
    Dynamic Communication Services
    20 Worman Lane
    Bernville, PA 19506
    Linda@DyComServ.com

ISBN-10:0615626718
ISBN-13: 978-061626710

Printed and manufactured in the United States of America
First Printing: 2012 CreateSpace

Table of Contents

PREFACE

<u>The Birth of the Partnership</u>
This book is finally being printed as the result of a chance "meeting" on the Dietetics in Health Care Communities (DHCC) Dietetic Practice Group (DPG) electronic mail list of the Academy of Nutrition and Dietetics between Digna and Linda.

Diane L Huth, RD, LDN, CDP has been a registered dietitian part time in LTC for almost 23 years. She posted the following email to the DHCC DPG electronic mail list:

> "Wondering what others are doing for fortified food diets: i.e. recipes you are
> using. How are you fortifying foods? I've gotten recipes from several
> sources. Just wondering what others are doing."

Digna responded, "I'm hoping to come out with a recipe manual for food fortification soon." Digna had worked on and off on this project for years and almost completed it in the summer of 2011. She had tested all the recipes for ease of prep as well as taste. However, the delay was always having the time to format and continue the publishing process.

Linda saw Digna's post and inquired: "Are you working on or planning to work on a fortified foods manual? If so, I have a collection of 25 high calorie, high protein drink recipes that I use for home hospice patients I'd be willing to share with you. These have worked great to provide variety. With the exception of Carnation Instant Breakfast, the shakes are made with "real food"." Linda published several books before and knew many of the items to consider for publication and marketing a book. This was the missing link to move Digna's book project forward. And so, the partnership began.

Having spent many years working as clinical dietitians in long-term care and/or hospice, we both bring a wealth of insight about the need for getting more nutrition into a smaller quantity of food without the use of commercial products. Making nutrient dense foods offers more variety and better intake for the nutritionally compromised individual.

We know there is a large market for this information – individuals receiving hospice and home care services; group homes, independent living, assisted living, and long-term care facilities; family members; Area Agency on Aging; dietary managers and dietitians. The recipes in this book are provided in portions for one and ten servings so they can be used at home or in a facility setting.

<u>Institutional Use Disclaimer</u>
Please be sure to check all regulations that apply to your institution regarding food preparation and food safety before using these recipes. Some ingredients may need to be altered to meet the regulations.

<u>Terminology</u>
There are many different terms used to identify the type of foods we are talking about in this book – enriched, fortified, nutrient-dense, and super. We are using the term fortified since we

are adding ingredients that will increase the amount of nutrients as well as provide additional calories.

How to Use This Book
The book is divided in to six common recipe categories – beverages; breads and cereals; desserts; main dishes; sauces and soups; and sides. Obviously missing are fruits and vegetables. Since fruits are used primarily in beverages to provide extra nutrition, look for fruits in the beverage section. Most of the time vegetables have a cream or cheese sauce added to increase the nutritional level. Check out the sauce and soup section of the book for more ideas.

The nutritional analysis is provided as a guide for professionals. Individuals consuming these recipes need all the nutrition they can get in a smaller quantity. However, we need to caution that a key to successful acceptance of a fortified food may not be the recipe with the most calories, protein or fat, but the recipe with ingredients that the individual enjoys eating so they consume more. Some nutrient values may vary based on the nutrient data available for products and specific items used in analysis. For example, the nutrition provided in the USDA products listed in the Nutritionist Pro SQL software may vary from a specific brand of an ingredient. Optional items and garnishes are not included in the nutritional analysis.

Each recipe provides ingredient quantities for both one and ten portions. However, there may be times that you want a different quantity than we have provided. Here are some simple guidelines to assist you to get the desired number of portions.
For:
  2 portions – use 2 times the 1 portion amounts
  3 portions – use 3 times the 1 portion amounts
  4 portions – use 4 times the 1 portion amounts
  5 portions – use half the 10 portion amounts

When the portion size is the same, recipe conversion factors can be determined by taking the number of portions you want and divide by the number of portions you have in the recipe. For example, you want 15 portions. By using the 10 portion information on the recipe (15 ÷ 10), your conversion factor is 1.5. This means you multiply each ingredient by 1.5 to determine the quantity of each ingredient needed for the 15 portions. If you have 10 portions and want 7 portions (7 ÷ 10), your conversion factor is 0.7. This means you multiply each ingredient by 0.7 to determine the quantity of each ingredient needed. Note that as yields are increased or decreased the cooking time will change.

Thanks and Acknowledgements

Thanks to:
- Diane L. Huth, RD LDN CDP for her post to the DHCC EML that got us together.
- Jessica C Beaudoin, RD for developing the recipe format and doing a lot of typing
- Derek Murphy of Creativindie Covers for the cover design
- Friends and colleagues for being our sounding board and dietary staff at Mesa Verde Convalescent Hospital for testing recipes
- Patients, residents, and clients who have tried the recipes over many years and enjoyed what they were eating and drinking
- Our reviewers Mascha A. Davis, MPH, RD; Marina Dobbie; Patty Keegan, RD; and Wayne Toczec

Temperature Guidelines

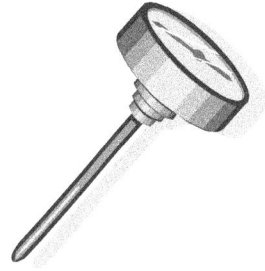

Cook foods to proper temperature

Foods are safely cooked when they are heated at a high enough temperature for a long enough time to kill disease causing organisms. The target temperature is different for different foods. Make sure that each food is cooked to the recommended temperature which ranges from 145° Fahrenheit (63° Celsius) to 165° Fahrenheit (74° Celsius).

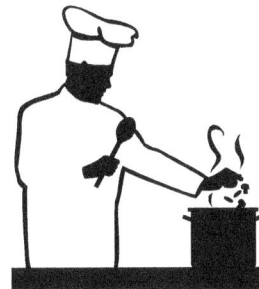

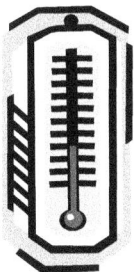

Cool foods promptly at proper temperature

Once food is prepared it should be eaten right away. Since cold temperatures slow the growth of bacteria, if you're saving it for later, cool rapidly in the refrigerator to 41° Fahrenheit (5° Celsius).

Proper thawing and reheating temperature

Thaw all frozen foods in the refrigerator and not at room temperature to avoid spoilage. When reheating be sure that the inside of the food reaches 165° Fahrenheit (74° Celsius) to be safe.

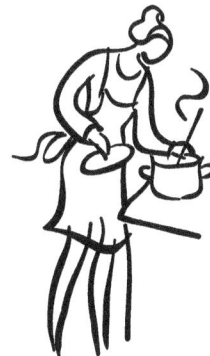

Beverages

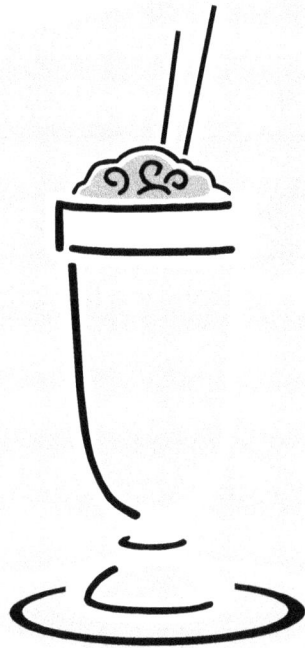

Apple Pie à la Mode Shake

Start to Finish: 10 min
Active Time: 10 min

Ingredients	1 Serving	10 Servings
Milk, whole	3 Tbsp	2 ¼ cup
Ice cream, vanilla	½ cup	4 ½ cups
Apple pie filling	½ cup	4 ½ cups

Method of Preparation

1. Blend all ingredients in a blender or food processor until smooth.

Nutrition Facts per 1 cup serving

Calories	Protein	Carbohydrates	Fat
298 kcal	4 g	52 g	9 g

Helpful Hints

* Garnish with a dash of cinnamon or whipped cream
* Use fortified milk to add more nutrition
* Use cherry pie filling for a cherry pie a la mode shake

Apricot Smoothie

Start to Finish: 10 min
Active Time: 10 min

Ingredients	1 Serving	10 Servings
Yogurt, vanilla or plain	¼ cup	2 ½ cups
Whole milk	¼ cup	2 ½ cups
Apricots in heavy syrup	½ cup	5 cups
Honey	3 ¼ tsp	⅔ cup

Method of Preparation

1. Blend all ingredients in a blender or food processor until smooth.

Nutrition Facts per 1 cup serving

Calories	Protein	Carbohydrates	Fat
244 kcal	6 g	52 g	3 g

Helpful Hints

* Garnish with whipped topping
* For variety, change the fruit or flavor of yogurt
* Use fortified milk to increase nutrition

Banana Nut Milkshake

Start to Finish: 10 min
Active Time: 10 min

Ingredients	1 Serving	10 Servings
Half and half	½ cup	5 cups
Ice cream, vanilla	¾ cup	2 quarts
Instant breakfast mix, vanilla	1 package	10 packages
Black walnut extract	1 capful	10 caps full
Banana, ripe	½ each	5 each

Method of Preparation

1. Blend all ingredients in a blender or food processor until smooth.

Nutrition Facts per 1 cup serving

Calories	Protein	Carbohydrates	Fat
543 kcal	13 g	69 g	25 g

Helpful Hints

* Garnish with crushed walnuts and sliced bananas
* Try different flavored ice creams, such as coffee or chocolate
* Try vanilla or banana yogurt or chocolate milk instead of half and half

Breakfast Shake

🕐 **Start to Finish:** 10 min
Active Time: 10 min

Ingredients

Ingredients	1 Serving	10 Servings
Milk, whole	½ cup	5 cups
Oatmeal, cooked and chilled	¼ cup	2 ½ cups
Banana, frozen	½ each	5 each
Wheat germ	1 ½ tsp	⅓ cup
Honey	1 ½ tsp	⅓ cup
Vanilla extract	½ tsp	4 tsp

Method of Preparation

1. Blend all ingredients in a blender or food processor until smooth.

Nutrition Facts per 1 cup serving

Calories	Protein	Carbohydrates	Fat
222 kcal	7 g	37 g	5 g

✧ Helpful Hints

* To garnish, sprinkle with cinnamon or top with sliced bananas
* Change fruit to strawberries or peaches for variety

Chocolate Almond Milkshake

Start to Finish: 10 min
Active Time: 10 min

Ingredients

Ingredients	1 Serving	10 Servings
Half and half	½ cup	5 cups
Ice cream, chocolate	¾ cup	2 quarts
Instant breakfast mix, chocolate	1 package	10 packages
Almond extract	½ capful	5 caps full

Method of Preparation

1. Blend all ingredients in a blender or food processor until smooth.

Nutrition Facts per 1 cup serving

Calories	Protein	Carbohydrates	Fat
575 kcal	14 g	55 g	33 g

Helpful Hints

* For an added protein boost, add peanut butter
* Variations can be made with chocolate milk, vanilla ice cream, or vanilla instant breakfast mix

Chocolate Cocoa Shake

Start to Finish: 10 min
Active Time: 10 min

Ingredients	1 Serving	10 Servings
Whole milk	½ cup	5 cups
Ice cream, vanilla	¾ cup	2 quarts
Hot chocolate mix	1 package	10 packages
Sugar	1 ½ tsp	⅓ cup

Method of Preparation

1. Blend all ingredients in a blender or food processor until smooth.

Nutrition Facts per 1 cup serving

Calories	Protein	Carbohydrates	Fat
528 kcal	10 g	68 g	25 g

◇ Helpful Hints

* Garnish with whipped topping or marshmallows
* Use chocolate milk and chocolate ice cream for a triple chocolate shake
* Use fortified milk or fortified chocolate milk to increase nutrition

Chocolate Peanut Butter Milkshake

Start to Finish: 10 min
Active Time: 10 min

Ingredients	1 Serving	10 Servings
Half and half	¼ cup	2 ½ cups
Ice cream, vanilla	1 cup	2 ½ quarts
Vanilla extract	½ tsp	5 tsp
Peanut butter	3 ¾ tsp	¾ cup
Chocolate syrup	4 ¾ tsp	1 cup

Method of Preparation

1. Blend all ingredients in a blender or food processor until smooth.

Nutrition Facts per 1 cup serving

Calories	Protein	Carbohydrates	Fat
564 kcal	12 g	57 g	33 g

✧ Helpful Hints

* Garnish with whipped topping and chocolate sauce or crushed peanut butter cup candies
* Vary the flavor by trying chocolate, peanut butter or banana ice cream or chocolate milk

Cinnamon Peach Smoothie

Start to Finish: 10 min
Active Time: 10 min

Ingredients	1 Serving	10 Servings
Yogurt, plain	¼ cup	2 ½ cups
Whole milk	¼ cup	2 ½ cups
Peaches, diced (frozen or canned)	½ cup	5 cups
Honey	1 ½ tsp	⅓ cup
Cinnamon	⅛ tsp	1 ¼ tsp

Method of Preparation

1. Blend all ingredients in a blender or food processor until smooth.

Nutrition Facts per 1 cup serving

Calories	Protein	Carbohydrates	Fat
202 kcal	6 g	41 g	3 g

Helpful Hints

* Garnish with whipped topping and cinnamon
* For variety try peach yogurt or change both the yogurt and fruit flavors

Classic Instant Breakfast Milkshake

Start to Finish: 10 min
Active Time: 10 min

Ingredients

Ingredients	1 Serving	10 Servings
Instant breakfast mix, any flavor	1 package	10 packages
Whole milk	½ cup	5 cups
Ice cream, vanilla	¾ cup	2 quarts

Method of Preparation

1. Blend all ingredients in a blender or food processor until smooth.

Nutrition Facts per 1 cup serving

Calories	Protein	Carbohydrates	Fat
409 kcal	12 g	56 g	15 g

◇ Helpful Hints

* Let your imagination run wild with flavor combinations by varying ice cream, instant breakfast, or milk flavors
* Use fortified milk to increase nutrition

Coffee Milkshake

Start to Finish: 10 min
Active Time: 10 min

Ingredients

Ingredients	1 Serving	10 Servings
Instant coffee	1 package	10 packages
Hot water	1 Tbsp	⅔ cup
Half and half	½ cup	5 cups
Ice cream, vanilla	¾ cup	2 quarts
Instant breakfast mix, vanilla	1 package	10 packages

Method of Preparation

1. Dissolve the instant coffee in hot water. Blend all ingredients in a blender or food processor until smooth.

Nutrition Facts per 1 cup serving

Calories	Protein	Carbohydrates	Fat
496 kcal	12 g	56 g	25 g

Helpful Hints

* Try this shake with chocolate ice cream for a mocha flavor or add flavored creamer
* Garnish with whipped topping or cinnamon

Cottage Cheese Smoothie

Start to Finish: 10 min
Active Time: 10 min

Ingredients	1 Serving	10 Servings
Cottage cheese	⅓ cup	3 ⅓ cup
Ice cream, vanilla	½ cup	5 cups
Flavored gelatin, ready to eat	¼ cup	2 ½ cups

Method of Preparation

1. Blend all ingredients in a blender or food processor until smooth.

Nutrition Facts per 1 cup serving

Calories	Protein	Carbohydrates	Fat
243 kcal	12 g	28 g	28 g

Helpful Hints

* Garnish with crushed walnuts and sliced bananas
* Try strawberry ice cream or orange sherbet for variety

| **Creamy Fruit Salad Shake** | | **Start to Finish:** | 10 min |
| | | **Active Time:** | 10 min |

Ingredients	1 Serving	10 Servings
Half and half	¼ cup	2 ½ cups
Whole milk	¼ cup	2 ½ cups
Cottage cheese	3 Tbsp	1 ⅔ cups
Fruit cocktail	⅓ cup	3 ⅓ cups
Liquid gelatin (any flavor)	3 Tbsp	1 ⅔ cups

Method of Preparation

1. Blend all ingredients in a blender or food processor until smooth.

Nutrition Facts per 1 cup serving

Calories	Protein	Carbohydrates	Fat
228 kcal	9 g	24 g	11 g

Helpful Hints

* Garnish with whipped topping and maraschino cherries
* For a pina colada spin, try this shake with pineapples and top with shaved coconut
* For additional variety, try tropical mixed fruit or other fruit combinations
* Replace half and half or cottage cheese with yogurt

Dairy-Free Citrus Cream Shake

Start to Finish: 10 min
Active Time: 10 min

Ingredients	1 Serving	10 Servings
Light corn syrup	¼ tsp	½ cup
Liquid non-dairy creamer	¼ cup	1 ½ quarts
Citrus powdered drink mix	¼ tsp	½ cup
Vegetable oil	1 tsp	¾ cup
Sherbet, citrus flavored	6 Tbsp	3 ½ cups

Method of Preparation

1. In a blender, combine the corn syrup, liquid non-dairy creamer, citrus flavored mix and oil, blend until smooth.
2. Add the sherbet, blend. Serve immediately.

Nutrition Facts per 1 cup serving

Calories	Protein	Carbohydrates	Fat
207 kcal	1 g	25 g	12 g

Helpful Hints

* For an extra protein boost, add protein powder
* Garnish with an orange slice
* If using a sugar-free powdered drink mix calories and carbohydrates will be less

Dairy-Free Coffee Latté

Start to Finish: 10 min
Active Time: 10 min

Ingredients	1 Serving	10 Servings
Water	¼ cup	2 ½ cups
Instant coffee powder	1 Tbsp	⅔ cup
Liquid non-dairy creamer	¾ cup	7 ½ cups
Sugar (optional)	3 Tbsp	2 cups

Method of Preparation

1. Bring water to a boil and remove from heat. Add instant coffee powder and sugar (optional), stirring until dissolved
2. Heat liquid non-dairy creamer to a simmer, stir in coffee syrup. Serve hot.

Nutrition Facts per 1 cup serving

Calories	Protein	Carbohydrates	Fat
234 kcal	1 g	23 g	15 g

Helpful Hints

* Prepare coffee syrup ahead of time and add to chilled non-dairy liquid creamer for a refreshing coffee drink
* Syrup can be stored for up to a week in the refrigerator
* For additional protein use soy milk in place of liquid non-dairy creamer
* Garnish hot or cold beverage with whipped topping and cinnamon or chocolate syrup
* If not intolerant to dairy products prepare coffee with half-and-half or evaporated milk
* If you have made coffee in the morning, save some in the refrigerator and use instead of water and instant coffee in this recipe

Dairy-Free Eggnog

Start to Finish: 10 min
Active Time: 10 min

Ingredients	1 Serving	10 Servings
Liquid non-dairy creamer	¾ cup	7 ½ cups
Eggs, liquid pasteurized	¼ cup	2 ½ cups
Sugar	2 Tbsp	1 ¼ cup
Vanilla extract	1 ¼ tsp	2 ½ Tbsp

Method of Preparation

1. In a saucepan or double boiler, combine liquid non-dairy creamer, liquid eggs, and sugar. Bring to a slow simmer, stirring. Remove from heat and add vanilla.
2. Chill eggnog in a shallow pan in the refrigerator. Serve chilled, with garnish of choice

Nutrition Facts per 1 cup serving

Calories	Protein	Carbohydrates	Fat
357 kcal	7g	48 g	15 g

✧ Helpful Hints

* Garnish eggnog with cinnamon, nutmeg, whipped topping, or chocolate syrup
* For an added protein boost, try using soy milk instead of non-dairy creamer. If using flavored milk substitute, omit vanilla and adjust sugar as needed
* Eggnog can be made with evaporated milk, if dairy able to tolerate dairy products
  o If using raw shell eggs be sure to cook eggs thoroughly: To make 1 serving 1 medium egg = ¼ cup, 10 servings 10 medium eggs = 2 ½ cups

Dairy-Free Shake

Start to Finish: 10 min
Active Time: 10 min

Ingredients	1 Serving	10 Servings
Sweetened soy milk	½ cup	5 cups
Soy yogurt	½ cup	5 cups
Banana, sliced	½ each	5 each
Wheat germ	3 ¼ tsp	⅔ cup
Protein powder	3 ¼ tsp	⅔ cup

Method of Preparation
1. Blend all ingredients in a blender or food processor until smooth.

Nutrition Facts per 1 cup serving

Calories	Protein	Carbohydrates	Fat
269 kcal	16 g	42 g	5 g

◇ Helpful Hints
* For an additional protein add peanut butter
* Variations can be made with flavored soy yogurt, soy milk, or different fresh or drained canned fruit

Fortified Milk

🕐 **Start to Finish:**   6 hr 5 min
Active Time: 5 min

Ingredients	1 Serving	10 Servings
Whole milk	1 cup	2 ½ quart
Non-fat dry milk	¼ cup	2 ½ cups

Method of Preparation
1. Blend ingredients, refrigerate for 6 hours

Nutrition Facts per 1 cup serving

Calories	Protein	Carbohydrates	Fat
257 kcal	19 g	27 g	8 g

✦ **Helpful Hints**
*   Fortified milk can also be made with any kind of milk - buttermilk, lactaid milk, chocolate milk
*   Add a flavored syrup or powder for variety, such as chocolate or strawberry

Fruit Shake

Start to Finish: 10 min
Active Time: 10 min

Ingredients	1 Serving	10 Servings
Whole milk	¼ cup	2 ½ cups
Ice cream, vanilla	¼ cup	2 ½ cups
Juice, apple, apricot, grape or peach	¾ cup	2 quarts
Vanilla extract	¼ tsp	2 ½ tsp

Method of Preparation

1. Blend all ingredients in a blender or food processor until smooth.

Nutrition Facts per 1 cup serving

Calories	Protein	Carbohydrates	Fat
193 kcal	3 g	32 g	6 g

Helpful Hints

* Garnish with sliced strawberries or other fruit
* In the summertime, add berries or fresh fruit to make a smoothie

Hawaiian Float Shake

Start to Finish: 10 min
Active Time: 10 min

Ingredients

Ingredients	1 Serving	10 Servings
Instant breakfast mix, vanilla	¼ package (1 T)	2 ½ packages
Evaporate whole milk	½ cup	5 cups
Orange-pineapple juice concentrate	2 Tbsp	1 ¼ cup
Ice water	¼ cup	2 ½ cups
Sherbet, lime	¼ cup	2 ½ cups

Method of Preparation

1. Blend all ingredients in a blender or food processor until smooth.

Nutrition Facts per 1 cup serving

Calories	Protein	Carbohydrates	Fat
311 kcal	11 g	44 g	10 g

◇ Helpful Hints

* Garnish with an orange slice
* Try this shake with raspberry or orange sherbet

High-Protein Milkshake

Start to Finish: 10 min
Active Time: 10 min

Ingredients	1 Serving	10 Servings
Whole milk	¼ cup	2 ½ cups
Non-fat dry milk	3 Tbsp	2 cups
Ice cream, vanilla	1 cup	10 cups

Method of Preparation

1. Blend all ingredients in a blender or food processor until smooth.

Nutrition Facts per 1 cup serving

Calories	Protein	Carbohydrates	Fat
392 kcal	15 g	46 g	17 g

◇ Helpful Hints

* Vary the flavor by substituting flavored ice cream for vanilla or using flavored milk
* Flavor the shake with chocolate syrup, smooth peanut butter, banana, or berries

Lemon Sherbet Shake

Start to Finish: 2 hr 10 min
Active Time: 10 min

Ingredients

Ingredients	1 Serving	10 Servings
Sugar	½ cup	5 cups
Lemon juice	4 ¾ tsp	1 cup
Lemon rind, grated	1 ½ tsp	⅓ cup
Whole milk	⅔ cup	6 ⅔ cup

Method of Preparation

1. Mix the sugar, juice, and rind in blender or food processor on high for 2 minutes. Slowly add in the milk.
2. Pour into a freezer tray and freeze. Cut into bite-sized pieces to serve.

Nutrition Facts per 1 cup serving

Calories	Protein	Carbohydrates	Fat
494 kcal	5 g	110 g	5 g

✧ Helpful Hints

* Garnish with a dash of cinnamon
* Orange or lime can be used to change the flavor

Mint Milkshake		Start to Finish:	10 min
		Active Time:	10 min

Ingredients

Ingredients	1 Serving	10 Servings
Half and half	½ cup	5 cups
Ice cream, vanilla	¾ cup	2 quarts
Instant breakfast mix, vanilla	1 package	10 packages
Peppermint extract	½ capful	5 caps full

Method of Preparation

1. Blend all ingredients in a blender or food processor until smooth.

Nutrition Facts per 1 cup serving

Calories	Protein	Carbohydrates	Fat
518 kcal	13 g	59 g	26 g

✧ Helpful Hints

* Garnish with whipped topping and fresh mint or chocolate sauce
* For a chocolate mint milkshake, use either chocolate ice cream or chocolate instant breakfast mix and mint extract
* Try making this shake with mint chocolate ice cream or chocolate milk for extra flavor

Peach Milkshake

Start to Finish: 10 min
Active Time: 10 min

Ingredients

Ingredients	1 Serving	10 Servings
Half and half	½ cup	5 cups
Ice cream, vanilla	½ cup	5 cups
Instant breakfast mix, vanilla	1 package	10 packages
Peaches canned halves	2 halves	20 halves

Method of Preparation

1. Blend all ingredients in a blender or food processor until smooth.

Nutrition Facts per 1 cup serving

Calories	Protein	Carbohydrates	Fat
528 kcal	12 g	75 g	21 g

Helpful Hints

* Garnish with crushed walnuts and sliced bananas
* Try different flavored ice creams, such as coffee, chocolate, or peach
* Change the fruit for even more variety
* Sliced peaches – ¾ cups = 2 halves

Peach Yogurt Frost

Start to Finish: 10 min
Active Time: 10 min

Ingredients	1 Serving	10 Servings
Instant breakfast mix, vanilla	½ package	5 packages
Whole milk	½ cup	5 cups
Yogurt, peach	¼ cup	2 ½ cups
Ice cubes, crushed	3-5 each	30-50 each

Method of Preparation

1. Blend all ingredients in a blender or food processor until smooth.

Nutrition Facts per 1 cup serving

Calories	Protein	Carbohydrates	Fat
199 kcal	8 g	31 g	5 g

✧ Helpful Hints

* Garnish with whipped topping and a maraschino cherry
* With so many yogurt flavor available, the sky is the limit for variety

Peanut Butter and Banana Milkshake

Start to Finish: 10 min
Active Time: 10 min

Ingredients

Ingredients	1 Serving	10 Servings
Whole milk	⅓ cup	3 ⅓ cups
Yogurt, plain	⅓ cup	3 ⅓ cups
Banana	1 each	10 each
Peanut butter, smooth	2 Tbsp	1 ¼ cups

Method of Preparation

1. Blend all ingredients in a blender or food processor until smooth.

Nutrition Facts per 1 cup serving

Calories	Protein	Carbohydrates	Fat
411 kcal	16 g	48 g	20 g

✧ Helpful Hints

* Garnish with crushed walnuts and sliced bananas
* Try different flavored ice creams such as peanut butter or chocolate
* Try banana yogurt or chocolate milk for additional variety

Peppermint Milkshake

Start to Finish: 10 min
Active Time: 10 min

Ingredients

Ingredients	1 Serving	10 Servings
Half and half	½ cup	5 cups
Ice cream, vanilla	¾ cup	2 quarts
Instant breakfast mix, vanilla	1 package	10 packages
Peppermint extract	½ to 1 capful	5-10 caps full
Red food coloring	2 drops	20 drops

Method of Preparation

1. Blend all ingredients in a blender or food processor until smooth.

Nutrition Facts per 1 cup serving

Calories	Protein	Carbohydrates	Fat
491 kcal	12 g	56 g	25 g

Helpful Hints

* Garnish with crushed or whole mini candy canes
* If you use peppermint ice cream, taste to determine if peppermint extract is desired

Rich Choco-Nutty Shake

Start to Finish: 10 min
Active Time: 10 min

Ingredients

Ingredients	1 Serving	10 Servings
Heavy whipping cream	2 Tbsp	1¼ cups
Ice cream, chocolate	⅔ cup	6⅔ cups
Peanut butter	3¼ tsp	⅔ cup
Chocolate syrup	3¼ tsp	⅔ cup

Method of Preparation

1. Blend all ingredients in a blender or food processor until smooth.

Nutrition Facts per 1 cup serving

Calories	Protein	Carbohydrates	Fat
502 kcal	10 g	37 g	36 g

Helpful Hints

* Garnish with whipped topping and chocolate syrup or crushed peanut butter cup candies
* For variety, use peanut butter ice cream or chocolate milk

Sherbet Shake

Start to Finish: 10 min
Active Time: 10 min

Ingredients	1 Serving	10 Servings
Whole milk	½ cup	5 cups
Sherbet	1 cup	10 cups
Vanilla extract	½ tsp	5 tsp

Method of Preparation
1. Blend all ingredients in a blender or food processor until smooth.

Nutrition Facts per 1 cup serving

Calories	Protein	Carbohydrates	Fat
294 kcal	5 g	51 g	7 g

◇ **Helpful Hints**
* Garnish with whipped topping
* For variety, change the flavor sherbet
* Use fortified milk to increase nutrition provided

Tropical CocoNog

Start to Finish: 10 min
Active Time: 10 min

Ingredients

Ingredients	1 Serving	10 Servings
Sweetened Condensed milk	¼ cup	2 cups
Evaporated milk	¼ cup	2 cups
Coconut cream	¼ cup	2 cups
Water	¼ cup	2 cups
Vanilla	To taste	To taste

Method of Preparation

1. Mix all ingredients until smooth. Serve cold

Nutrition Facts per 1 cup serving

Calories	Protein	Carbohydrates	Fat
366 kcal	6 g	53 g	15 g

Helpful Hints

* Garnish with cinnamon or nutmeg
* Use pineapple juice instead of water for a piña colada
* Ingredients can also be mixed in a blender or food processor

Breads and Cereals

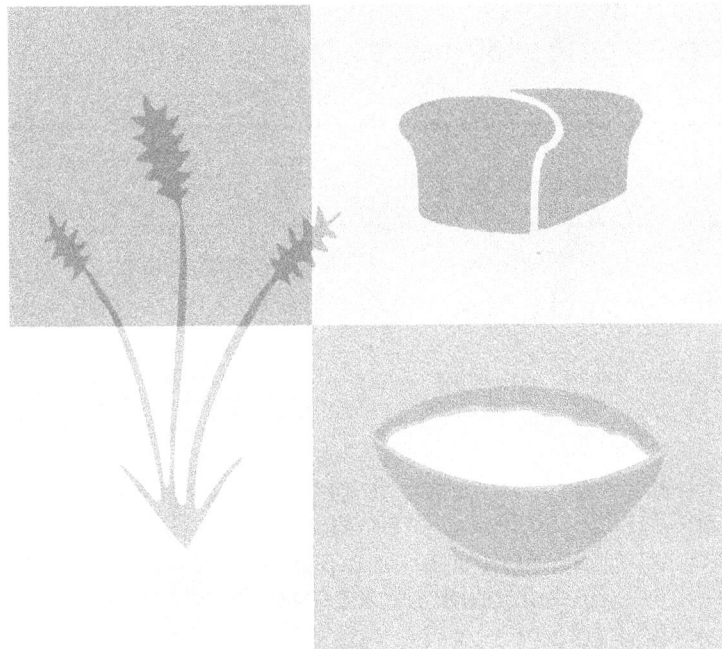

Baked Dressing Casserole

Start to Finish: 45 min
Active Time: 15 min

Ingredients	1 Serving	10 Servings
Bread	1 slice	10 slices
Margarine	2 ½ tsp	½ cup
Condensed Cream soup, undiluted	¼ cup	3 cups
Seasoning, any type	To taste	To taste

Method of Preparation

1. Preheat oven to 350°F. Break bread into cubes, about 1 inch. Place bread into a pan with deep enough sides.
2. Heat cream soup. Combine margarine and soup, add seasoning to taste. Drizzle evenly over bread cubes, stir to coat.
3. Bake dressing for 15 to 30 minutes, until golden brown.

Nutrition Facts per ½ cup serving

Calories	Protein	Carbohydrates	Fat
201 kcal	3 g	18 g	13 g

✧ Helpful Hints

* Seasoning ideas: garlic powder, oregano and basil; onion powder, cilantro, and chili powder; poultry seasoning blend
* Baked Dressing Casserole can be made with any type of bread, such as whole wheat, French bread, cornbread, or biscuits
* The size portion depends on the type of bread used and the size and density of the slice. To measure accurately divide the finished recipe into 10 equal portions

Breakfast Bread Pudding

Start to Finish: 45 min
Active Time: 15 min

Ingredients	1 Serving	10 Servings
Bread, cubed	1 slice	10 slices
Evaporated milk	⅓ cup	1 quart
Eggs , beaten	1 each	5 each
Margarine, melted	2 ½ tsp	½ cup
Sugar	2 ½ tsp	½ cup
Cinnamon	Dash	1 tsp
Nutmeg	Dash	1 tsp
Cloves, powdered	Dash	1 tsp

Method of Preparation

1. Preheat oven to 350°F. Cut bread into cubes, about 1 inch. Place bread in a greased baking dish.
2. Combine evaporated milk, eggs, melted margarine, sugar and spices in a bowl and mix until well-combined. Pour mixture over bread and stir to moisten bread thoroughly.
3. Bake for 30 minutes, until a knife inserted in the center comes out clean. Serve hot or cold.

Nutrition Facts per ½ cup serving

Calories	Protein	Carbohydrates	Fat
370 kcal	12 g	34 g	21 g

Helpful Hints

* Garnish with honey, melted jam or cinnamon if served hot; or if served cold, garnish with whipped topping, powdered sugar or cinnamon
* Bread pudding can be made with day-old bread, croissants, whole wheat bread, or sweet rolls
* The size portion depends on the type of bread used and the size and density of the slice. To measure accurately divide the finished recipe into 10 equal portions
* 1 slice cubed sandwich bread makes a scant ½ cup dry, 1/3 cup soaked
* A dash is also a pinch, less than 1/8 tsp, or to taste

Dairy-free Super Cereal

Start to Finish: 30 min
Active Time: 30 min

Ingredients

Ingredients	1 Serving	10 Servings
Hot cereal, dry	3 tbsp	2 cups
Liquid non-dairy creamer	⅓ cup	6 cups
Eggs, liquid pasteurized	4¾ tsp	1 cup
Margarine	4¾ tsp	1 cup

Method of Preparation

1. Mix liquid non-dairy creamer with dry hot cereal in a sauce pan. Cook stirring constantly to avoid lumps until thickened..
2. Slowly temper the eggs then add them back into the hot cereal slowly over low heat, stirring constantly.
3. Heat to 160°F, stirring constantly. Add margarine, stir until melted.

Nutrition Facts per 1 cup serving

Calories	Protein	Carbohydrates	Fat
409 kcal	5 g	29 g	31 g

◇ Helpful Hints

* Add raisins, brown sugar, crushed nuts, honey, maple syrup, black strap molasses, or any other toppings
* Thin with additional creamer if desired.
* For a protein boost use soy milk instead of non-dairy creamer
* If using shell eggs whip to mix then measure. When making one portion may refrigerate the remaining portion of egg for use within 24 hours as an ingredient or freeze for later use.
* If not dairy-intolerant may substitute evaporated milk or half-and-half for non-dairy creamer
* To temper the eggs:
  * Mix the hot cereal mixture into the eggs, whisking to mix. Continue adding until about 1/3 of hot the hot cereal has been incorporated into eggs, Slowly return eggs-hot cereal mixture to the hot cereal pot, stirring to mix well. Keep the fire low to prevent scorching.

Enriched Cereal

Start to Finish: 30 min
Active Time: 30 min

Ingredients	1 Serving	10 Servings
Hot cereal, dry	½ cup	5 cups
Evaporated milk	1 cup	2½ quarts
Non-fat dry milk	2 Tbsp	1¼ cups
Margarine	4 ¾ tsp	1 cup

Method of Preparation

1. Mix evaporated milk and non-fat dry milk. Mix in dry hot cereal..
2. Cook over low heat stirring constantly to avoid lumps or sticking until thickened.
3. Add margarine, stir until melted.

Nutrition Facts per 1 cup serving

Calories	Protein	Carbohydrates	Fat
709 kcal	28 g	61 g	40 g

Helpful Hints

* May serve with Super Topping, raisins, brown sugar, crushed nuts, honey, maple syrup, black strap molasses, or any of your favorite fruits

Desserts

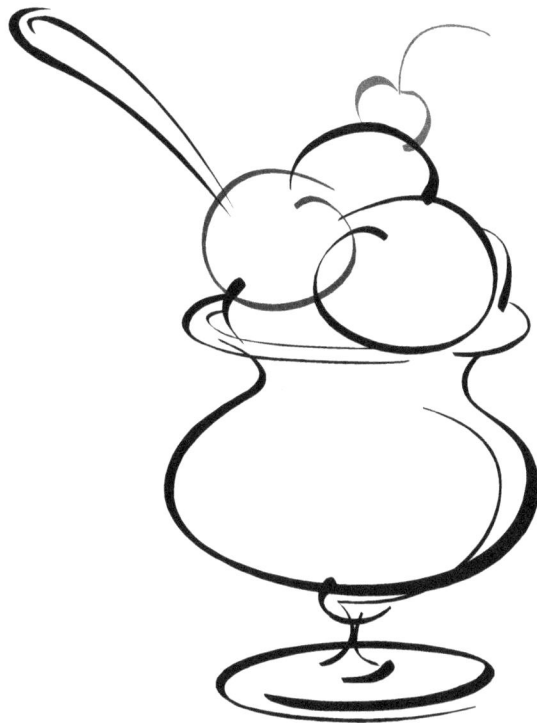

Ambrosia

Start to Finish: 2 hr 15 min
Active Time: 15 min

Ingredients

Ingredients	1 Serving	10 Servings
Sweetened condensed milk	3 Tbsp	2 cups
Lemon juice	2 ½ tsp	½ cup
Canned mixed fruit, drained	¼ cup	3 cups
Corn syrup, light	1 ¼ tsp	¼ cup
Whipped topping	4 ¾ tsp	1 cup

Method of Preparation

1. Combine condensed milk and lemon juice, allow to stand and thicken for 5 minutes.
2. Stir in the fruit and corn syrup, then fold in whipped topping.
3. Chill covered for 2 hours in the refrigerator, or for 30 to 45 minutes in the freezer.

Nutrition Facts per ½ cup serving

Calories	Protein	Carbohydrates	Fat
289 kcal	5 g	54 g	7 g

✧ Helpful Hints

* Garnish with flaked coconut or mini marshmallows
* Vary the recipe by trying different canned fruits, such as a tropical mix or peaches and pears

Fruited Gelatin

Ingredients	1 Serving	10 Servings
Fruit, canned, drained, pureed	¼ cup	2 ½ cups
Juice from can + water to make	4 ¾ tsp	1 cup
Flavored gelatin	4 ¾ tsp	1 cup
Evaporated milk	4 ¾ tsp	1 cup
Lemon juice	½ tsp	4 tsp

Method of Preparation

1. Drain fruit, reserving liquid in measuring cup. Add water to the amount indicated to make the desired portion. Bring to a boil, remove from heat.
2. Mix gelatin with hot liquid stirring until dissolved. Add the evaporated milk and mix well. Stir in the pureed fruit and lemon juice.
3. Chill gelatin until firm. Garnish as desired.

Nutrition Facts per ½ cup serving

Calories	Protein	Carbohydrates	Fat
163 kcal	4 g	33 g	2 g

Helpful Hints

* Use your favorite fruits or applesauce
* Avoid high fiber fruits that may not puree well and high acid fruits such as orange or fresh pineapple that may prevent gelatin from setting up
* Garnish with whipped topping and a small piece of the fruit used in the filling
* Try varying the gelatin flavors with strawberry, orange, tropical fruit, or lime

Peanut Butter Cup Pudding

Start to Finish: 1 hr 20 min
Active Time: 20 min

Ingredients	1 Serving	10 Servings
Prepared pudding, chocolate	2 Tbsp	1 ¼ cup
Peanut butter, creamy	4 ¾ tsp	1 cup
Evaporated milk	4 ¾ tsp	1 cup
Vegetable oil	3 ¾ tsp	¾ cup
Chocolate syrup	2 Tbsp	1 ¼ cup

Method of Preparation
1. Prepare the pudding according to directions on the box.
2. Combine all ingredients in a blender or mixer, or mix by hand in a bowl.
3. Chill the pudding mixture in the refrigerator for at least one hour.

Nutrition Facts per ½ cup serving

Calories	Protein	Carbohydrates	Fat
478 kcal	10 g	40 g	33 g

Helpful Hints
* Pudding can be stored in the refrigerator for up to three days
* Garnish pudding with chocolate chips, a dollop of jam, sliced bananas, or sprinkles
* Add some texture by using crunchy peanut butter or crushed peanuts
* Try different flavored puddings for variety, such as vanilla or banana cream

Peanut Butter Frosting

🕐 **Start to Finish:** 30 min
Active Time: 30 min

Ingredients

Ingredients	1 Serving	10 Servings
Margarine, softened	1 ¼ tsp	¼ cup
Powdered sugar	2 tsp	6 Tbsp
Peanut butter	1 tsp	3 Tbsp
Vanilla extract	Drops	¼ tsp
Liquid non-dairy creamer	Drops	¼ tsp

Method of Preparation

1. In a mixer, whip softened margarine. Slowly add powdered sugar. Add the peanut butter, vanilla and creamer. Whip until smooth and creamy.

Nutrition Facts per 1 Tbsp serving

Calories	Protein	Carbohydrates	Fat
86 kcal	1 g	5 g	7 g

◇ **Helpful Hints**

* Spread peanut butter frosting over muffins, brownies, sugar cookies, cakes, or between graham crackers
* Frosting can be stored for up to one week in the refrigerator

Rice Pudding

Start to Finish: 2 hr 20 min
Active Time: 20 min

Ingredients	1 Serving	10 Servings
Margarine, melted	1 ¼ tsp	¼ cup
Cottage cheese	3 Tbsp	2 cups
Sugar	1 ¼ tsp	¼ cup
Salt	⅛ tsp	1½ tsp
Vanilla	⅛ tsp	1½ tsp
Raisins	¼ tsp	1 Tbsp
Cooked rice	3 Tbsp	2 cups
Eggs, liquid pasteurized	3 ¾ tsp	¾ cup
Evaporated milk	2 ½ tsp	½ cup

Method of Preparation

1. Preheat oven to 350°F. Combine melted margarine, cottage cheese, sugar, salt, vanilla, raisins and cooked rice. Mix thoroughly.
2. Combine eggs and evaporated milk, then fold into rice.
3. Spread rice mixture in a greased baking dish, bake until a knife inserted in the center comes out clean, about 20 minutes.
4. Serve rice pudding hot, or chill in the refrigerator and serve cold.

Nutrition Facts per ½ cup serving

Calories	Protein	Carbohydrates	Fat
384 kcal	17 g	35 g	19 g

◇ Helpful Hints

* Garnish with a sprinkle of cinnamon, a small fruit wedge, top with whipped topping, soft jam or chocolate syrup
* If using shell eggs whip to mix before measuring. When making one portion, refrigerate the remaining portion of egg for use within 24 hours as an ingredient or freeze for later use. 1 medium egg = ¼ cup

Super Pudding

Start to Finish: 1 hr 15 min
Active Time: 15 min

Ingredients	1 Serving	10 Servings
Whole milk	3 Tbsp	2 cups
Evaporated milk	3 Tbsp	2 cups
Corn syrup, light	3 ¾ tsp	¾ cup
Vegetable oil	1 ¼ tsp	¼ cup
Pudding, instant, any flavor	¾ ounce	7 ounces
Non-fat dry milk	4 ¾ tsp	1 cup

Method of Preparation
1. Combine whole and evaporated milks, corn syrup and vegetable oil.
2. Add the instant pudding and non-fat dry milk and mix well.
3. Pour the pudding mixture into a dish and cover. Chill in the refrigerator for at least one hour.

Nutrition Facts per ½ cup serving

Calories	Protein	Carbohydrates	Fat
318 kcal	7 g	50 g	11 g

Helpful Hints
* Garnish with whipped topping, chocolate syrup, chocolate chips, marshmallows, crushed nuts, a dollop of jelly, or fruit
* Pudding can be stored for up to one week in the refrigerator

Main Dishes

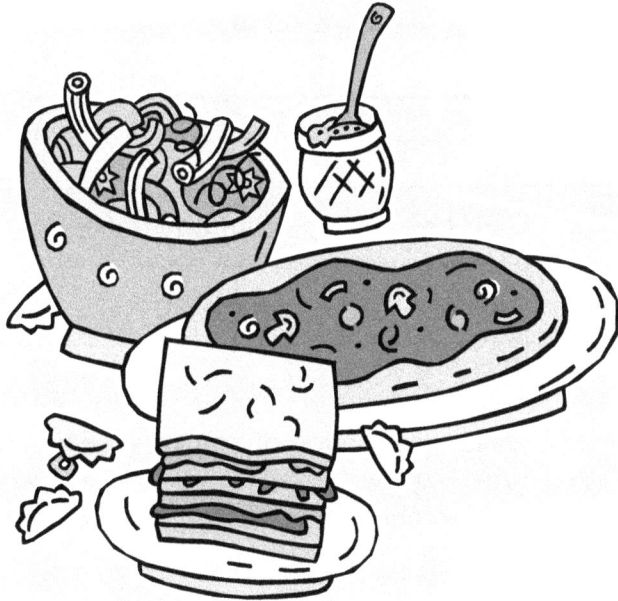

Egg Salad

Start to Finish: 40 min
Active Time: 15 min

Ingredients	1 Serving	10 Servings
Mayonnaise	2 ½ tsp	½ cup
Evaporated milk	2 ½ tsp	½ cup
Mustard	¼ tsp	2 tsp
Eggs, hard cooked, cooled, chopped	1 each	10 each
Celery, diced (optional)	1 ¼ tsp	¼ cup
Onion, diced (optional)	1 ¼ tsp	¼ cup

Method of Preparation

1. In a bowl, mix mayonnaise, evaporated milk and mustard.
2. Stir in the hard cooked eggs, celery and onions if using. Chill the egg salad for about 25 minutes before serving.

Nutrition Facts per ¾ cup serving

Calories	Protein	Carbohydrates	Fat
141 kcal	7 g	5 g	10 g

✧ Helpful Hints

* Serve egg salad over lettuce, on top of crackers, or on toasted bread for a sandwich
* For variety, add shredded cheese, crumbled bacon, pickle relish, or diced tomatoes

Hearty Meat Stew	Start to Finish:	40 min
	Active Time:	15 min

Ingredients	1 Serving	10 Servings
Sour cream	4 ¾ tsp	1 cup
Evaporated milk	¼ cup	2 ½ cup
Cooked beef, diced	3 ounces	2 pounds
Gravy	¼ cup	2 ½ cup

Method of Preparation
1. In a saucepan combine sour cream and evaporated milk, add gravy.
2. Stir in meat. Bring the stew to a slow simmer on the stove, stirring frequently. Season to taste.

Nutrition Facts per 1 cup serving

Calories	Protein	Carbohydrates	Fat
324 kcal	26 g	11 g	19 g

◇ **Helpful Hints**
 * Hearty stew can also be made using chicken, pork, or turkey
 * Add cooked vegetables, such as carrots, peas, potatoes, celery, onions, and/or tomatoes for a complete meal
 * Use the Rich Gravy recipe for even more calories and a rich flavor

Savory Meatloaf

Start to Finish: 1 hr 20 min
Active Time: 20 min

Ingredients	1 Serving	10 Servings
Evaporated milk	3 ¾ tsp	¾ cup
Eggs, beaten	3 ¾ tsp	3 each
Non-fat dry milk	2 ½ tsp	½ cup
Oatmeal	2 Tbsp	1 ½ cup
Garlic powder	Dash	Dash
Pepper	To taste	To taste
Ground beef	4 ounces	2 ½ pounds
Cheese, shredded	2 ½ tsp	½ cup
Onion, chopped	2 ½ tsp	½ cup
Celery, chopped	2 ½ tsp	½ cup

Method of Preparation

1. Combine evaporated milk, eggs, and non-fat dry milk. Stir in oatmeal, garlic powder and pepper.
2. Add egg mixture to ground beef, add cheese, onion, and celery. Mix.
3. For 10 servings: Divide mixture into loaves and bake in cookie sheet at at 350°F for 1 to 1 ½ hours or until internal temperature in the center reaches 165°F.
4. For an individual serving: Form meatloaf into a patty and bake on a small sheet pan or cook in frying pan for 10 – 15 minutes

Nutrition Facts per 4 ounce serving

Calories	Protein	Carbohydrates	Fat
309 kcal	20 g	7 g	22 g

✧ Helpful Hints

* Serve meatloaf with gravy, barbecue sauce, or hearty tomato sauce
* Try topping meatloaf with ketchup or barbeque sauce before baking
* Substitute ground turkey for ground beef

Savory Meat Soufflé

Start to Finish: 1 hr 20 min
Active Time: 20 min

Ingredients

Ingredients	1 Serving	10 Servings
Cooked beef	3 ounces	2 pounds
Evaporated milk	¼ cup	2 ½ cups
Eggs, liquid pasteurized	2 Tbsp	1 ½ cups
Onion powder	¼ tsp	2 ½ tsp
Garlic powder	¼ tsp	2 ½ tsp

Method of Preparation

1. Preheat oven to 350°F.
2. In a food processor, grind meat until smooth, add evaporated milk and eggs. If mixture is too dry, add more evaporated milk.
3. Pour mixture into a greased pan and bake until the internal temperature in the center reaches 165°F, about 30 minutes. Cut into squares and serve with gravy or sauce of choice.

Nutrition Facts per ¾ cup serving

Calories	Protein	Carbohydrates	Fat
292 kcal	34 g	8 g	14 g

✧ Helpful Hints

* Meat soufflé can be made with beef, chicken, turkey, fish, ham, pork or turkey
* Vary flavors by using your preferred herbs and spices mix
* Serve meat soufflé with gravy, a dollop of sour cream, barbecue sauce, fresh chopped herbs or parmesan cheese
* Try meat soufflé as a cold sandwich with sliced tomatoes, lettuce, onions, and mayonnaise
* If using shell eggs whip to mix then measure. When making one portion, refrigerate the remaining portion of egg for use within 24 hours as an ingredient or freeze for later use. 1 medium egg = ¼ cup.

Tuna Salad

Start to Finish: 40 min
Active Time: 15 min

Ingredients

Ingredients	1 Serving	10 Servings
Mayonnaise	2 ½ tsp	½ cup
Evaporated milk	2 ½ tsp	½ cup
Mustard	¼ tsp	2 tsp
Tuna, drained	½ cup	5 cups
Hard-cooked eggs, chopped	1	10
Celery, diced	1 tbsp	1 ¼ cups
Pepper	To taste	To taste

Method of Preparation

1. In a bowl, mix mayonnaise, evaporated milk and mustard.
2. Mix the drained tuna with chopped egg, celery and pepper.
3. Pour in the mayonnaise dressing and toss to coat salad well.
4. Chill for about 1 hour before serving.

Nutrition Facts per ¾ cup serving

Calories	Protein	Carbohydrates	Fat
232 kcal	27 g	5 g	11 g

✧ Helpful Hints

* Serve tuna salad over lettuce, on top of crackers, or on toasted bread for a sandwich
* For additional crunch try adding diced sweet red peppers, chopped onions or scallions, pickle relish
* A dash of oregano flakes and garlic powder add an interesting taste
* Try adding crumbled bacon, sunflower seeds, or sliced green olives
* For a hot treat make a sandwich adding a slice of your preferred cheese and grill until the bread is toasted and the cheese melts

Sauces and Soups

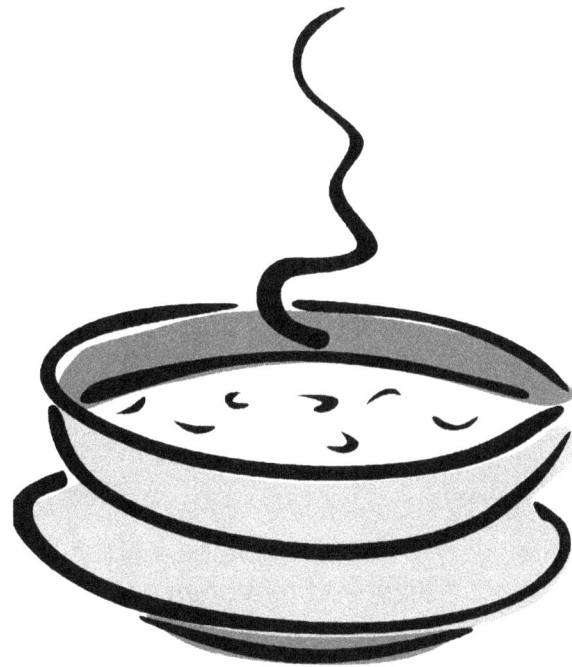

Rich Gravy

Start to Finish: 30 min
Active Time: 30 min

Ingredients	1 Serving	10 Servings
Gravy mix	2 ½ tsp	½ cup
Hot water	1 ¼ Tbsp	1 ¼ cups
Non-fat dry milk	2 Tbsp	1 ½ cup
Liquid non-dairy creamer	3 Tbsp	2 cups
Margarine, melted	2 ½ tsp	½ cup

Method of Preparation
1. In a saucepan, stir the gravy mix into the hot water until free of lumps.
2. Over low-medium heat, stir in the non-fat dry milk, non-dairy creamer, melted margarine.
3. Bring the gravy to a slow simmer, stirring constantly to prevent scorching.

Nutrition Facts per 1/3 cup serving

Calories	Protein	Carbohydrates	Fat
227 kcal	7 g	17 g	15 g

Helpful Hints
* Serve with meat, poultry, mashed potatoes, or biscuits
* Prepare gravy ahead of time, and reheat as needed. Store for up to one week in the refrigerator
* To reheat the gravy, place in a saucepan and warm over low-medium heat, stirring constantly until bubbly

Super Topping

Start to Finish: 20 min
Active Time: 20 min

Ingredients	1 Serving	10 Servings
Margarine, melted	3 ¾ tsp	¾ cup
Evaporated milk	3 Tbsp	2 cups
Non-fat dry milk	3 ¾ tsp	¾ cup
Brown sugar	3 ¾ tsp	¾ cup

Method of Preparation

1. In a saucepan, combine margarine, evaporated milk, non-fat dry milk and brown sugar.
2. Bring to a slow simmer, stirring constantly, for about 15 minutes.

Nutrition Facts per ¼ cup serving

Calories	Protein	Carbohydrates	Fat
270 kcal	5 g	24 g	17 g

Helpful Hints

* Serve super topping with hot cereal, French toast, pancakes or bran muffins
* Pour ¼ cup of this topping over sliced or diced canned or fresh fruits and bake until hot and bubbly for a delicious and easy dessert
* Try flavoring super topping with cloves, cinnamon, or nutmeg

51

Bean Soup

Start to Finish: 50 min
Active Time: 10 min

Ingredients	1 Serving	10 Servings
Margarine	4 ¾ tsp	1 cup
Onions, chopped	1 ¼ tsp	¼ cup
Celery, diced	3 Tbsp	2 cups
Canned beans, drained	¼ cup	3 cups
Ham or other deli meat, diced	2 ½ tsp	½ cup
Non-fat dry milk	4 ¾ tsp	1 cup
Evaporated milk	3 Tbsp	2 cups
Broth, chicken, beef or vegetable	½ cup	5 cups
Pepper	To taste	To taste

Method of Preparation

1. In a saucepan, melt the margarine. Sauté the celery and onion over medium heat until tender, about 10 minutes.
2. Add the beans and ham to the saucepan, bring to a simmer.
3. Mix non-fat dry milk with evaporated milk stirring to dissolve. Add the broth, and milk mixture, stir to combine. Simmer for 30 minutes.
4. Adjust seasoning if needed.

Nutrition Facts per 1 cup serving

Calories	Protein	Carbohydrates	Fat
354 kcal	15 g	25 g	23 g

Helpful Hints

* Try black beans, navy beans, lentils, kidney beans, or a combination of beans for more variety
* Use a variety of herbs to season such as cumin, oregano, parsley or chili powder
* Garnish with parmesan cheese, shredded cheese, crumbled crisp bacon, a dollop of sour cream, plain yogurt or fresh herbs.

Cheddar Cheese Soup

Start to Finish: 1 hr 30 min
Active Time: 30 min

Ingredients	1 Serving	10 Servings
Margarine	2 ½ tsp	½ cup
Onion, chopped	1 ¼ tsp	¼ cup
Broth, chicken	6 Tbsp	1 quart
Evaporated milk	6 Tbsp	1 quart
Worcestershire sauce	¼ tsp	2 tsp
Cheddar cheese, mild or sharp, grated	6 Tbsp	1 quart

Method of Preparation

1. Melt margarine. Cook the onions until translucent. Add chicken broth and evaporated milk.
2. Bring to a high simmer on medium heat. Add Worcestershire sauce and cheddar cheese. Stir until cheese is completely melted.

Nutrition Facts per 1 cup serving

Calories	Protein	Carbohydrates	Fat
402 kcal	17 g	13 g	31 g

✧ Helpful Hints

* Garnish soup with croutons, chopped vegetables, chives, paprika, sour cream or plain yogurt
* Try making cheddar soup with Tabasco sauce, chili powder or cayenne for an added kick
* Prepare soup with vegetables or potatoes for a more complete meal

Chunky Potato Chowder

Start to Finish: 2 hr 10 min
Active Time: 40 min

Ingredients	1 Serving	10 Servings
Margarine	1 tsp	⅓ cup
Onions, chopped	¾ tsp	3 Tbsp
Flour	¾ tsp	3 Tbsp
Salt	⅛ tsp	1 ½ tsp
Pepper	Dash	Dash
Cooked potatoes, diced	¼ cup	2 ½ cups
Non-fat dry milk	2 Tbsp	1 ½ cup
Evaporated milk	⅔ cup	1 ½ quarts

Method of Preparation

1. In a soup pot, melt margarine and sauté onions until translucent, about 10 minutes.
2. Add flour, salt, and pepper to onions, cook over medium heat stirring to prevent scorching or lumping for about 2 to 3 minutes.
3. Mix the non-fat dry milk with evaporated milk and heat. Slowly add milk mixture to the onion and flour mixture.
4. Add the cooked potatoes. Heat to a slow simmer stirring occasionally to prevent scorching and until it thickens.
5. Adjust seasonings if necessary.

Nutrition Facts per 1 cup serving

Calories	Protein	Carbohydrates	Fat
353 kcal	18 g	33 g	17 g

✧ Helpful Hints

* Garnish soup with chopped parsley, parmesan cheese, a dollop of sour cream or plain yogurt, or crumbled bacon
* If necessary may add milk or broth to thin
* Try making potato chowder with bacon fat instead of margarine
* Make different types of chowder by adding corn, canned clams, or diced ham

Cream Soup Base

Start to Finish: 25 min
Active Time: 25 min

Ingredients	1 Serving	10 Servings
Margarine	4 ¾ tsp	1 cup
Flour	4 ¾ tsp	1 cup
Salt	Dash	1 tsp
Powdered milk	4 ¾ tsp	1 cup
Broth	6 Tbsp	1 quart
Evaporated milk	½ cup	1 ½ quarts
White pepper	To taste	To taste

Method of Preparation

1. Melt margarine in a sauté pan, whisk in flour and salt. Stir to a smooth consistency, and cook until toasty but not browned.
2. In a saucepan, combine powdered milk, broth and evaporated milk, bring to a slow simmer.
3. Slowly add milk mixture to the flour and margarine. Stir frequently to avoid scorching, cook until thickened. Season with white pepper.

Nutrition Facts per 1 cup serving

Calories	Protein	Carbohydrates	Fat
461 kcal	17 g	32 g	30 g

◇ Helpful Hints

* Cream soup base can be used as a cream sauce for meats or vegetables, or as a base four creamy soups
* Try the following varieties of cream soup: carrots, broccoli, corn, mushrooms, asparagus or cauliflower

Jiffy Enriched Soup

Start to Finish: 30 min
Active Time: 30 min

Ingredients	1 Serving	10 Servings
Whole milk	⅓ cup	3 ¼ cups
Evaporated milk	5 Tbsp	2- 12 oz cans
Non-fat dry milk	3 ¾ tsp	¾ cup
Cream soup, condensed	¼ cup	2- 10.5 oz cans

Method of Preparation

1. In a bowl, combine whole milk, evaporated milk and non-fat dry milk until non-fat dry milk is dissolved.
2. Place cream soup in a saucepan, slowly add the milk mixture. Heat to a slow simmer and serve.

Nutrition Facts per 1 cup serving

Calories	Protein	Carbohydrates	Fat
230 kcal	12 g	21 g	11 g

◇ Helpful Hints

* Try making the soup with cream of tomato, cream of mushroom , cream of chicken, cream of celery, cream of broccoli, or cream of potato soup
* Garnish soup with chopped herbs, shredded cheese, sour cream or a pat of butter

56

Lentil Soup

Start to Finish: 1 hr 30 min
Active Time: 30 min

Ingredients	1 Serving	10 Servings
Lentils, dry	1 ounce	12 ounces
Water	⅔ cup	1 ½ quart
Onions, chopped	1½ tsp	⅓ cup
Celery, chopped	1½ tsp	⅓ cup
Carrots, sliced	3 ¾ tsp	¾ cup
Bay leaf	½ each	1 each
Salt	To taste	1 tsp
Pepper	Dash	Dash
Nutmeg	Dash	Dash
Non-fat dry milk	2 ½ tsp	½ cup
Broth	4 ¾ tsp	1 cup
Half and half	3 Tbsp	2 cups

Method of Preparation

1. Wash lentils with cold water, drain. In a saucepan, bring lentils and water to a boil. Add the chopped vegetables and bay leaf and stir in seasonings
2. Simmer, covered, for 1 hour or until vegetables and lentils are tender. Remove the bay leaf.
3. Mix the non-fat dry milk with the broth and add half and half.
4. Pour into the lentil mixture and bring back to a simmer before serving.

Nutrition Facts per 1 cup serving

Calories	Protein	Carbohydrates	Fat
215 kcal	13 g	28 g	6 g

✦ Helpful Hints

* Garnish soup with chopped herbs, sour cream, a drizzle of olive oil, diced ham or scallions
* If desired, evaporated milk can be substituted for half and half

Pizzazz Pumpkin Soup

Start to Finish: 1 hr 30 min
Active Time: 30 min

Ingredients	1 Serving	10 Servings
Non-fat dry milk	3 ¾ tsp	¾ cup
Water	4 ¾ tsp	1 cup
Cream soup, condensed	½ cup	3- 10.5 oz can
Evaporated milk	5 Tbsp	2- 12 oz cans
Margarine	1 ¼ tsp	¼ cup
Onion, chopped	3 ½ tsp	⅔ cup
Pumpkin, canned	¼ cup	3 cups
Nutmeg	Dash	⅛ tsp
Tabasco sauce (optional)	Dash	1 tsp

Method of Preparation

1. Dissolve non-fat dry milk into the water in a bowl. Add the soup, and evaporated milk. Heat to a simmer.
2. In a sauté pan, melt the margarine and sauté the onions until translucent. Add onions to the soup mixture.
3. Add pumpkin and nutmeg, stir until combined. Simmer for about 10 minutes and serve.

Nutrition Facts per 1 cup serving

Calories	Protein	Carbohydrates	Fat
275 kcal	11 g	26 g	15 g

✧ Helpful Hints

* Garnish soup with chopped herbs, sour cream, a drizzle of olive oil, diced ham or scallions or onions, or a drizzle of honey
* For even more pizzazz may add chili powder or cayenne

Side Dishes

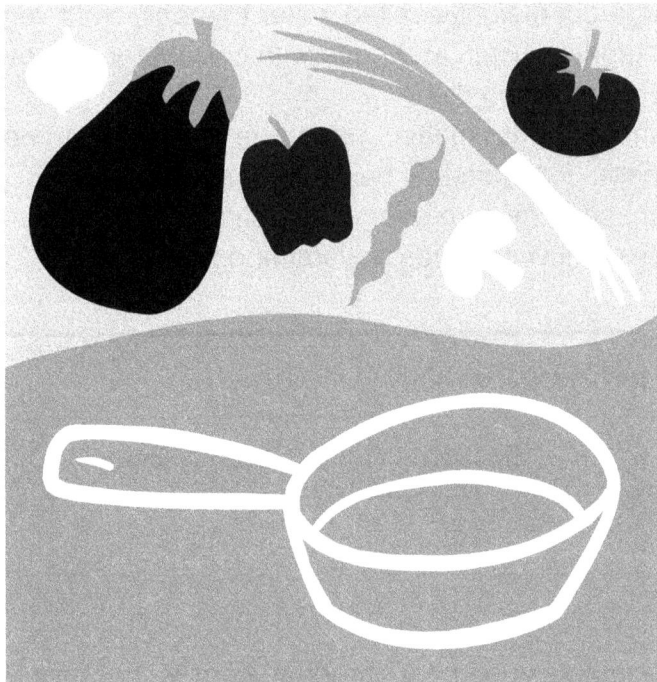

Creamed Vegetables

Start to Finish: 1 hr 25 min
Active Time: 25 min

Ingredients	1 Serving	10 Servings
Vegetables, shredded, lightly packed	⅔ cup	1 ½ quart
Condensed cream soup	¼ cup	2 ½ cups
Margarine, melted	2 ½ tsp	½ cup
Parsley flakes, dried	Dash	½ tsp
Basil, dried	Dash	¼ tsp
Pepper	To taste	¼ tsp

Method of Preparation

1. Preheat the oven to 350°F.
2. Bring a large pot of lightly salted water to a boil. Add vegetables and cook until tender. Drain and rinse with cold water to prevent carryover cooking. Put in baking dish.
3. Heat cream soup with melted margarine to a slow simmer in a saucepan over low heat. Add parsley, basil, and pepper.
4. Pour cream soup mixture over vegetables, toss to coat. Bake for 30 to 45 minutes, until vegetables are soft and browned.

Nutrition Facts per ½ cup serving

Calories	Protein	Carbohydrates	Fat
184 kcal	3 g	16 g	12 g

✧ Helpful Hints

* Vary the vegetables used: try shredded carrots, cabbage, peppers, mushrooms, celery or squash
* Garnish vegetables with parmesan cheese, diced herbs or try baking the vegetables with shredded cheese on top
* For a crunchy top, sprinkle with breadcrumbs before baking
* If using fresh herbs double the amount
* For convenience, use frozen or fresh packaged shredded vegetables

Creamy Pasta

Start to Finish: 1 hr 25 min
Active Time: 25 min

Ingredients	1 Serving	10 Servings
Cooked pasta	¼ cup	3 cups
Evaporated milk	4 ¾ tsp	1 cup
Margarine, melted	4 ¾ tsp	1 cup
Cottage cheese	¼ cup	3 cups
Parmesan cheese, grated	3 ¾ tsp	¾ cup
Garlic powder	¼ tsp	2 ½ tsp
Pepper	To taste	To taste

Method of Preparation

1. Preheat the oven to 350° F.
2. Cook pasta according to directions, drain and set aside.
3. In a bowl, combine all other ingredients and fold into the cooked pasta making sure it is not mashed or broken.
4. Spoon pasta mixture into a greased baking dish, and bake for 20 minutes or until cottage cheese is melted.

Nutrition Facts per ½ cup serving

Calories	Protein	Carbohydrates	Fat
355 kcal	14 g	19 g	25 g

Helpful Hints

* Garnish creamy pasta with fresh chopped basil, chopped sundried tomatoes, parmesan cheese, springs of chives or diced bacon
* For a crunchy and flavorful topping sprinkle with seasoned breadcrumbs

Creamy Vegetable Soufflé

Start to Finish: 1 hr
Active Time: 30 min

Ingredients	1 Serving	10 Servings
Margarine	¾ tsp	2 Tbsp
Onions, chopped	1 ¼ tsp	¼ cup
Frozen diced vegetables, thawed	2 oz	2- 10 oz bags
Eggs, liquid pasteurized	3 ¾ tsp	¾ cup
Sour cream	¼ cup	2 ½ cups
Condensed cream soup	¼ cup	2 ½ cups
Pepper	Dash	¼ tsp
Garlic powder	Dash	¼ tsp
Cheddar cheese, grated	4 ¾ tsp	1 cup

Method of Preparation
1. Preheat the oven to 350˚F.
2. Melt the margarine in a pan, sauté the onions until translucent.
3. In a bowl, mix together eggs, sour cream, condensed soup, pepper, garlic powder, and ¾ of the cheese. Add the onions and margarine used to sauté. Fold in the thawed vegetables
4. Spoon into a greased baking dish. Sprinkle the rest of the cheese on top. Bake for 20 to 30 minutes, until lightly set.

Nutrition Facts per ½ cup serving

Calories	Protein	Carbohydrates	Fat
363 kcal	10 g	21 g	25 g

✧ Helpful Hints
* Vary the vegetables used: try broccoli (diced after thawing), cut green beans, mixed vegetables or peas
* Try different cheeses, such as parmesan cheese, Pepper Jack, Swiss or provolone
* May also use fresh packaged shredded vegetables.
* If using shell eggs whip to mix then measure. When making one portion, refrigerate the remaining portion of egg for use within 24 hours as an ingredient or freeze for later use. 1 medium egg = ¼ cup

Mashed Potatoes

Start to Finish: 40 min
Active Time: 25 min

Ingredients	1 Serving	10 Servings
Evaporated milk	3 Tbsp	2 cups
Margarine	4 ¾ tsp	1 cup
Instant mashed potatoes	2 Tbsp	1 ½ cups
Pepper	To taste	To taste
Cottage cheese	4 ¾ tsp	1 cup

Method of Preparation
1. Heat evaporated milk and margarine to a slow simmer then turn off heat.
2. Stir in the instant mashed potatoes and pepper, mixing thoroughly until all flakes are moistened. If too dry add more evaporated milk to moisten.
3. Return the mashed potato mixture to the stove on a very low heat or double boiler to prevent scorching.
4. Stir in cottage cheese vigorously to prevent sticking. Cook until cottage cheese melts.

Nutrition Facts per ½ cup serving

Calories	Protein	Carbohydrates	Fat
278 kcal	7 g	12 g	23 g

◇ Helpful Hints
* Top mashed potatoes with a dollop of sour cream, shredded cheese, chives, paprika, or a spoonful of gravy
* For a soufflé- like texture spoon mashed potatoes into a greased baking dish and bake for 15 minutes at 350° F.

Mashed Sweet Potatoes

Start to Finish: 1 hr 15 min
Active Time: 45 min

Ingredients	1 Serving	10 Servings
Evaporated milk	3 Tbsp	2 cups
Margarine	4 ¾ tsp	1 cup
Salt	¼ tsp	1 Tbsp
Ground nutmeg	dash	2 tsp
Sweet potatoes, cooked and mashed	6 Tbsp	1 quart
Cottage cheese	4 ¾ tsp	1 cup
Eggs, liquid pasteurized	2 ½ tsp	½ cup

Method of Preparation
1. Preheat the oven to 300°F.
2. Heat evaporated milk and margarine to a slow simmer. Remove from heat. Stir in salt and nutmeg.
3. Combine mashed sweet potatoes, cottage cheese and eggs in a bowl, mixing thoroughly.
4. Slowly add the milk mixture to the sweet potato mixture.
5. Pour into a greased baking dish and bake for 45 minutes to 1 hour.

Nutrition Facts per ½ cup serving

Calories	Protein	Carbohydrates	Fat
371 kcal	9 g	30 g	25 g

✧ Helpful Hints
* Use canned sweet potatoes in place of fresh cooked sweet potatoes
* Garnish sweet potatoes with, chopped herbs or a dash of nutmeg
* Prepare sweet potatoes with brown sugar or maple syrup, or garnish with marshmallows before baking for a sweeter side dish
* If you like it hot add chili powder or cayenne to taste
* If using shell eggs whip to mix then measure. When making one portion refrigerate the remaining portion of egg for use within 24 hours as an ingredient or freeze for later use. One medium egg = ¼ cup

Savory Rice

Start to Finish: 1 hr 25 min
Active Time: 25 min

Ingredients	1 Serving	10 Servings
Cooked white rice	¼ cup	3 cups
Evaporated milk	4 ¾ tsp	1 cup
Cottage cheese	¼ cup	3 cups
Margarine	4 ¾ tsp	1 cup
Salt	¼ tsp	1 Tbsp
Pepper	To taste	To taste

Method of Preparation
1. Preheat the oven to 350°F.
2. In a bowl mix all ingredients.
3. Spoon mixture into a greased baking dish and bake for 20 minutes or until cottage cheese is melted. Stir and serve hot.

Nutrition Facts per ½ cup serving

Calories	Protein	Carbohydrates	Fat
323 kcal	11 g	18 g	23 g

◇ Helpful Hints
* Garnish with fresh chopped herbs
* Serve with a spoonful of gravy, a dash of reduced sodium soy sauce, or flavor the rice with herbs and seasonings before baking

Vegetable Au Gratin

Start to Finish: 1 hr
Active Time: 30 min

Ingredients	1 Serving	10 Servings
Vegetables, washed and sliced	3 Tbsp	4 cups
Condensed cream soup	¼ cup	2 ½ cups
Cheddar cheese, grated	2 Tbsp	1 ½ cups
Pepper	Dash	¼ tsp

Method of Preparation
1. Preheat the oven to 350°F.
2. Bring a pot of lightly salted water to a boil. Cook vegetables, covered, for 10 to 15 minutes or until tender. Drain and place in a baking dish.
3. Pour cream soup over vegetables, fold in cheese and pepper. Cover with foil, bake for 10 to 15 minutes until heated through.

Nutrition Facts per ½ cup serving

Calories	Protein	Carbohydrates	Fat
147 kcal	6 g	12 g	8 g

Helpful Hints
* Vary the vegetables used: try carrots, cauliflower, potatoes, peas, mushrooms, onions, summer squash or any combination
* Garnish with chopped herbs, parmesan cheese or sour cream
* If using shell eggs whip to mix then measure. When making one portion may refrigerate the remaining portion of egg for use within 24 hours as an ingredient or freeze for later use. 1 medium egg = ¼ cup, 8 – 10 medium eggs = 1 cup

Flavorful Fortified Foods – Recipes to Enrich Life

Recipe Index

Flavorful Fortified Food – Recipes to Enrich Life

Ingredient Index

Flavorful Fortified Food – Recipes to Enrich Life

Ingredient Index

- ✦ Mayonnaise – **44, 48**
- ✦ Milk, evaporated – **20, 30, 33, 35, 38, 39, 41, 42, 44, 45, 46, 47, 48, 51, 52, 53, 54, 55, 56, 58, 61, 63, 64, 65**
- ✦ Milk, non-fat dry – **18, 21, 35, 42, 46, 50, 51, 52, 54, 55, 56, 57, 58**
- ✦ Milk, sweetened condensed – **30, 37**
- ✦ Milk, whole - **2, 3, 5, 7, 9, 10, 13, 18, 19, 21, 22, 25, 26, 29, 42, 56**
- ✦ Mustard – **44, 48**
- ✦ Non-Dairy Creamer, liquid – **14, 15, 16, 34, 40, 50**
- ✦ Nutmeg, ground – **33, 57, 58, 64**
- ✦ Oatmeal, dry – **5, 46**
- ✦ Oil, vegetable – **14, 39, 42**
- ✦ Onion – **46, 52, 53, 54, 57, 58, 62**
- ✦ Onion Powder – **47**
- ✦ Parmesan Cheese, grated – **61**
- ✦ Parsley, dry flakes – **60**
- ✦ Pasta – **61**
- ✦ Peaches, frozen or canned – **9, 24**
- ✦ Peanut Butter – **8, 26, 28, 39, 40**
- ✦ Peppermint Extract – **23, 27**
- ✦ Potatoes - **54**
- ✦ Potatoes, instant mashed – **63**
- ✦ Protein Powder - **17**
- ✦ Pudding Mix – **39, 42**
- ✦ Pumpkin, canned – **58**
- ✦ Raisins – **41**
- ✦ Rice – **41, 65**
- ✦ Sherbet – **14, 20, 29**
- ✦ Sour Cream – **45, 62**
- ✦ Soy Milk – **17**
- ✦ Soy Yogurt - **17**
- ✦ Sugar, granulated – **7, 16, 22, 33, 41**
- ✦ Sugar, powdered – **40**
- ✦ Sugar, brown – **51**
- ✦ Sweet Potatoes - **64**
- ✦ Tuna, canned – **48**
- ✦ Vanilla Extract – **5, 8, 16, 19, 29, 40, 41**
- ✦ Vegetables, fresh or frozen – **60, 62, 66**
- ✦ Walnut Extract - **4**
- ✦ Wheat Germ – **5, 17**
- ✦ Whipped Topping – **37**
- ✦ Worcestershire Sauce – **53**
- ✦ Yogurt – **3, 9, 25, 26**

About the Authors

Digna Cassens, MHA, RD is the president of Cassens Associates – Diversified Nutrition Management System, providing consulting and management services to long-term care, assisted living and group homes, and medical nutritional therapy services for homebound clients. She completed a BS in Foods & Nutrition at Barry University; dietetic internship at Charity Hospital is New Orleans, and a Masters degree in Healthcare Administration from University of La Verne.

Digna specializes in food safety, sanitation, and project management. She has worked in long-term care for over 30 years and has experience in middle and senior management while working for some of the largest national public and private long-term care companies. She has developed specialties in cost effective menu design, budgetary compliance, and policy and procedure development. Digna is a legal forensic consultant specializing in medical nutrition therapy, nutrition and hydration, pressure areas, abuse and neglect. She has been a community college instructor and holds lifetime teaching credentials in California; has supervised and been a preceptor to dietetic interns; and developed and conducted English and Spanish language classes for dietary students and dietary supervisors.

Digna is a member of the Academy of Nutrition and Dietetics; the California Dietetic Association; Nutrition Entrepreneurs and Dietetics in Healthcare Communities Dietetic Practice Groups; and Latinos and Hispanics in Dietetics and Nutrition (LAHIDAN), a Member Interest Group. She has reviewed professional publications and books for the Academy and independent authors, worked on national and state level annual meetings, and volunteered as an appointed board member of DHCC. 2012 marks Digna's golden anniversary as a Registered Dietitian.

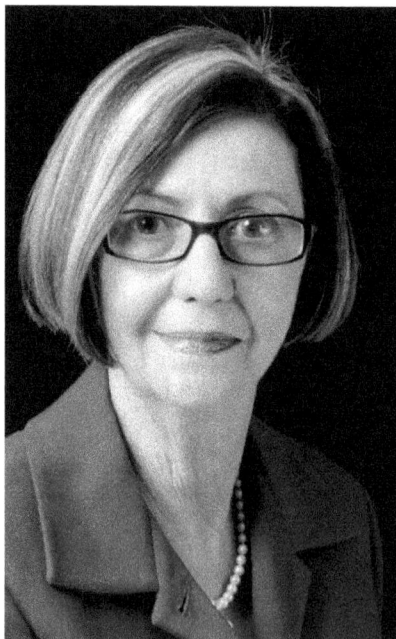

About the Authors

Linda S. Eck Mills, MBA, RD, FADA is the owner of Dynamic Communication Services where she is an international speaker, career and life coach, and author. She holds a BS in Home Economics Education from Mansfield University, MBA in Administrative Management from St Joseph's University, completed the Core Essentials Coaching Program from Coach U, and is a charter Fellow of the American Dietetic Association.

During her 30 years as a dietitian, Linda's work has included teaching dietetic, dietary manager, and hotel restaurant management courses; providing medical nutrition therapy in long-term care, an adolescent residential treatment center, corrections, hospice, and home care; ServSafe instructor; food service management; consulting; and food service equipment and food sales. She is the author of over 180 articles and 4 books, including *From Mundane to Ah Ha! Effective Training Objects* © 2005. She is a contributor *The 2010 Pfeiffer Annual: Consulting* © 2010; *The Leadership Challenge activities book* © 2010; *2009 Pfeiffer Annual: Training* © 2009; *Nutrition: Real People Real Choices* © 2009; *Trainer's Warehouse Book of Game* © 2008.

Linda is licensed in multiple states and is a member of a number of professional organizations including: Academy of Nutrition and Dietetics; Pennsylvania Dietetic Association; Dietetics in Health Care Communities, Nutrition Entrepreneurs, and Dietitians in Business and Communication Dietetic Practice Groups; Dietetic Practice Group sub-units for Coaches, Speakers, Authors, and Corrections; Association of Correctional Food Service Affiliates; the local chapter of ASTD (American Society for Training & Development); and has been a member of the National Speakers Association. She is the recipient of the Outstanding Dietitian in Pennsylvania Award and the Innovator Award from the Central Pennsylvania Dietetic Association.

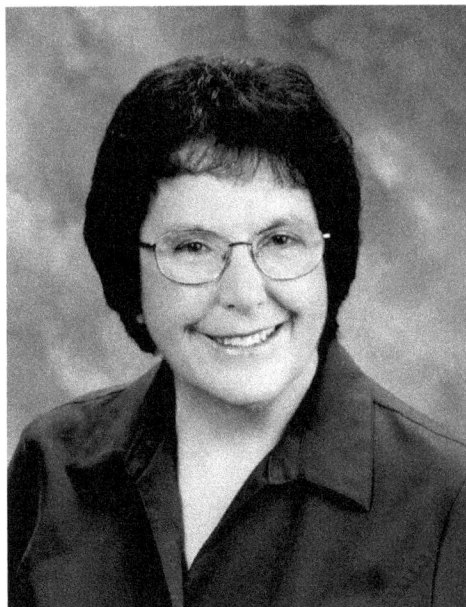

Complimentary Resources

Institutional users and care givers may order complimentary resources. The following training programs are available <u>directly from Digna Cassens, MHA, RD</u> at: dignacassens@gmail.com, or, PO Box 581, La Habra, CA 90633.

FREE when ordering single copies:
- Fortified Foods Program Lesson Plan , Syllabus and Competency Test
- Institutional storage time and temperature and HACCP guidelines

FREE when ordering 10 or more copies: The above <u>plus</u>
- Food fortification policy featuring individualized sample meal plans

FREE when ordering 50 or more copies: The above <u>plus</u>
- Fortified Foods Program Power Point presentation

The training programs are also available on CD for $15.00 per order directly from Digna Cassens

FREE 30 minute phone tele-conference with Digna Cassens, MHA, RD (by appointment) to answer questions and assist in providing additional staff training.

Submit the form below to dignacassens@gmail.com to request any of the above complimentary resources.

First Name	Last Name		Credentials
Company Name			
Email Address			
Address: Street, Number, City, State, Zip Code , Country		Business Phone	
		Other Phone	
List other book topics or training materials you may be interested in			
Are you interested in Kindle or electronic editions of this or similar books?		Y	N

www.ingramcontent.com/pod-product-compliance
Lightning Source LLC
Chambersburg PA
CBHW051418200326

41520CB00023B/7276